# ON ANCIENT MEDICINE

## Hippocrates of Kos
### *Father of Medicine*

**Translated:** Francis Adams
**Edited by:** D.P. Curtin

Dalcassian
Publishing
Company
PHILADELPHIA, PA

Library of Congress Cataloging-in-Publication Data

# Part I

Whoever having undertaken to speak or write on Medicine, have
first laid down for themselves some hypothesis to their argument,
such as hot, or cold, or moist, or dry, or whatever else they choose
(thus reducing their subject within a narrow compass, and supposing
only one or two original causes of diseases or of death among
mankind), are all clearly mistaken in much that they say; and this is
the more reprehensible as relating to an art which all men avail
themselves of on the most important occasions, and the good
operators and practitioners in which they hold in especial honor. For
there are practitioners, some bad and some far otherwise, which, if
there had been no such thing as Medicine, and if nothing had been
investigated or found out in it, would not have been the case, but all
would have been equally unskilled and ignorant of it, and everything
concerning the sick would have been directed by chance. But now it
is not so; for, as in all the other arts, those who practise them differ
much from one another in dexterity and knowledge, so is it in like
manner with Medicine. Wherefore I have not thought that it stood in
need of an empty hypothesis, like those subjects which are occult
and dubious, in attempting to handle which it is necessary to use
some hypothesis; as, for example, with regard to things above us and
things below the earth; if any one should treat of these and undertake
to declare how they are constituted, the reader or hearer could not
find out, whether what is delivered be true or false; for there is
nothing which can be referred to in order to discover the truth.

# Part II

But all these requisites belong of old to Medicine, and an origin and
way have been found out, by which many and elegant discoveries
have been made, during a length of time, and others will yet be
found out, if a person possessed of the proper ability, and knowing
those discoveries which have been made, should proceed from them
to prosecute his investigations. But whoever, rejecting and despising
all these, attempts to pursue another course and form of inquiry, and
says he has discovered anything, is deceived himself and deceives
others, for the thing is impossible. And for what reason it is
impossible, I will now endeavor to explain, by stating and showing
what the art really is. From this it will be manifest that discoveries
cannot possibly be made in any other way. And most especially, it

appears to me, that whoever treats of this art should treat of things which are familiar to the common people. For of nothing else will such a one have to inquire or treat, but of the diseases under which the common people have labored, which diseases and the causes of their origin and departure, their increase and decline, illiterate persons cannot easily find out themselves, but still it is easy for them to understand these things when discovered and expounded by others. For it is nothing more than that every one is put in mind of what had occurred to himself. But whoever does not reach the capacity of the illiterate vulgar and fails to make them listen to him, misses his mark. Wherefore, then, there is no necessity for any hypothesis.

## Part III

For the art of Medicine would not have been invented at first, nor would it have been made a subject of investigation (for there would have been no need of it), if when men are indisposed, the same food and other articles of regimen which they eat and drink when in good health were proper for them, and if no others were preferable to these. But now necessity itself made medicine to be sought out and discovered by men, since the same things when administered to the sick, which agreed with them when in good health, neither did nor do agree with them. But to go still further back, I hold that the diet and food which people in health now use would not have been discovered, provided it had suited with man to eat and drink in like manner as the ox, the horse, and all other animals, except man, do of the productions of the earth, such as fruits, weeds, and grass; for from such things these animals grow, live free of disease, and require no other kind of food. And, at first, I am of opinion that man used the same sort of food, and that the present articles of diet had been discovered and invented only after a long lapse of time, for when they suffered much and severely from strong and brutish diet, swallowing things which were raw, unmixed, and possessing great strength, they became exposed to strong pains and diseases, and to early deaths. It is likely, indeed, that from habit they would suffer less from these things then than we would now, but still they would suffer severely even then; and it is likely that the greater number, and those who had weaker constitutions, would all perish; whereas the stronger would hold out for a longer time, as even nowadays some, in consequence of using strong articles of food, get off with little trouble, but others with much pain and suffering. From this necessity it appears to me that they would search out the food befitting their nature, and thus discover that which we now use: and that from wheat, by macerating it, stripping it of its hull, grinding it all down, sifting, toasting, and baking it, they formed bread; and from barley they formed cake (maza), performing many operations in regard to it; they boiled, they roasted, they mixed, they diluted those things which are strong and of intense qualities with weaker things, fashioning them to the nature and powers of man, and considering that the stronger things Nature would not be able to manage if administered, and that from such things pains, diseases, and death would arise, but such as Nature could manage, that from them food, growth, and health, would arise. To such a discovery and investigation what more suitable name could one give than that of Medicine? since it was discovered for the health of man, for his nourishment and safety, as a substitute for that kind of diet by which pains, diseases, and deaths were occasioned.

## Part IV

And if this is not held to be an art, I do not object. For it is not suitable to call any one an artist of that which no one is ignorant of, but which all know from usage and necessity. But still the discovery is a great one, and requiring much art and investigation. Wherefore those who devote themselves to gymnastics and training, are always making some new discovery, by pursuing the same line of inquiry, where, by eating and drinking certain things, they are improved and grow stronger than they were.

## Part V

Let us inquire then regarding what is admitted to be Medicine; namely, that which was invented for the sake of the sick, which possesses a name and practitioners, whether it also seeks to accomplish the same objects, and whence it derived its origin. To me, then, it appears, as I said at the commencement, that nobody would have sought for medicine at all, provided the same kinds of diet had suited with men in sickness as in good health. Wherefore, even yet, such races of men as make no use of medicine, namely, barbarians, and even certain of the Greeks, live in the same way when sick as when in health; that is to say, they take what suits their appetite, and neither abstain from, nor restrict themselves in anything for which they have a desire. But those who have cultivated and invented medicine, having the same object in view as those of whom I formerly spoke, in the first place, I suppose, diminished the quantity of the articles of food which they used, and this alone would be sufficient for certain of the sick, and be manifestly beneficial to them, although not to all, for there would be some so affected as not to be able to manage even small quantities of their usual food, and as such persons would seem to require something weaker, they invented soups, by mixing a few strong things with much water, and thus abstracting that which was strong in them by dilution and boiling. But such as could not manage even soups, laid them aside, and had recourse to drinks, and so regulated them as to mixture and quantity, that they were administered neither stronger nor weaker than what was required.

## Part VI

But this ought to be well known, that soups do not agree with certain persons in their diseases, but, on the contrary, when administered both the fevers and the pains are exacerbated, and it becomes obvious that what was given has proved food and increase to the disease, but a wasting and weakness to the body. But whatever persons so affected partook of solid food, or cake, or bread, even in small quantity, would be ten times and more decidedly injured than those who had taken soups, for no other reason than from the strength of the food in reference to the affection; and to whomsoever it is proper to take soups and not eat solid food, such a one will be much more injured if he eat much than if he eat little, but even little food will be injurious to him. But all the causes of the sufferance refer themselves to this rule, that the strongest things most especially and decidedly hurt man, whether in health or in disease.

## Part VII

What other object, then, had he in view who is called a physician, and is admitted to be a practitioner of the art, who found out the regimen and diet befitting the sick, than he who originally found out and prepared for all mankind that kind of food which we all now use, in place of the former savage and brutish mode of living? To me it appears that the mode is the same, and the discovery of a similar nature. The one sought to abstract those things which the constitution of man cannot digest, because of their wildness and intemperature, and the other those things which are beyond the powers of the affection in which any one may happen to be laid up. Now, how does the one differ from the other, except that the latter admits of greater variety, and requires more application, whereas the former was the commencement of the process?

## Part VIII

And if one would compare the diet of sick persons with that of persons in health, he will find it not more injurious than that of healthy persons in comparison with that of wild beasts and of other animals. For, suppose a man laboring under one of those diseases which are neither serious and unsupportable, nor yet altogether mild, but such as that, upon making any mistake in diet, it will become apparent, as if he should eat bread and flesh, or any other of those articles which prove beneficial to healthy persons, and that, too, not in great quantity, but much less than he could have taken when in good health; and that another man in good health, having a constitution neither very feeble, nor yet strong, eats of those things which are wholesome and strengthening to an ox or a horse, such as vetches, barley, and the like, and that, too, not in great quantity, but much less than he could take; the healthy person who did so would be subjected to no less disturbance and danger than the sick person who took bread or cake unseasonably. All these things are proofs that Medicine is to be prosecuted and discovered by the same method as the other.

## Part IX

And if it were simply, as is laid down, that such things as are stronger prove injurious, but such as are weaker prove beneficial and nourishing, both to sick and healthy persons, it were an easy matter, for then the safest rule would be to circumscribe the diet to the lowest point. But then it is no less mistake, nor one that injuries a man less, provided a deficient diet, or one consisting of weaker things than what mare proper, be administered. For, in the constitution of man, abstinence may enervate, weaken, and kill. And there are many other ills, different from those of repletion, but no less dreadful, arising from deficiency of food; wherefore the practice in those cases is more varied, and requires greater accuracy. For one must aim at attaining a certain measure, and yet this measure admits neither weight nor calculation of any kind, by which it may be accurately determined, unless it be the sensation of the body; wherefore it is a task to learn this accurately, so as not to commit small blunders either on the one side or the other, and in fact I would give great praise to the physician whose mistakes are small, for perfect accuracy is seldom to be seen, since many physicians seem to me to be in the same plight as bad pilots, who, if they commit mistakes while conducting the ship in a calm do not expose themselves, but when a storm and violent hurricane overtake them, they then, from their ignorance and mistakes, are discovered to be what they are, by all men, namely, in losing their ship. And thus bad and commonplace physicians, when they treat men who have no serious illness, in which case one may commit great mistakes without producing any formidable mischief (and such complaints occur much more frequently to men than dangerous ones): under these circumstances, when they commit mistakes, they do not expose themselves to ordinary men; but when they fall in with a great, a strong, and a dangerous disease, then their mistakes and want of skill are made apparent to all. Their punishment is not far off, but is swift in overtaking both the one and the other.

## Part X

And that no less mischief happens to a man from unseasonable depletion than from repletion, may be clearly seen upon reverting to the consideration of persons in health. For, to some, with whom it agrees to take only one meal in the day, and they have arranged it so accordingly; whilst others, for the same reason, also take dinner, and this they do because they find it good for them, and not like those persons who, for pleasure or from any casual circumstance, adopt the one or the other custom and to the bulk of mankind it is of little consequence which of these rules they observe, that is to say, whether they make it a practice to take one or two meals. But there are certain persons who cannot readily change their diet with impunity; and if they make any alteration in it for one day, or even for a part of a day, are greatly injured thereby. Such persons, provided they take dinner when it is not their wont, immediately become heavy and inactive, both in body and mind, and are weighed down with yawning, slumbering, and thirst; and if they take supper in addition, they are seized with flatulence, tormina, and diarrhea, and to many this has been the commencement of a serious disease, when they have merely taken twice in a day the same food which they have been in the custom of taking once. And thus, also, if one who has been accustomed to dine, and this rule agrees with him, should not dine at the accustomed hour, he will straightway feel great loss of strength, trembling, and want of spirits, the eyes of such a person will become more pallid, his urine thick and hot, his mouth bitter; his bowels will seem, as it were, to hang loose; he will suffer from vertigo, lowness of spirit, and inactivity,- such are the effects; and if he should attempt to take at supper the same food which he was wont to partake of at dinner, it will appear insipid, and he will not be able to take it off; and these things, passing downwards with tormina and rumbling, burn up his bowels; he experiences insomnolency or troubled and disturbed dreams; and to many of them these symptoms are the commencement of some disease.

## Part XI

But let us inquire what are the causes of these things which happened to them. To him, then, who was accustomed to take only one meal in the day, they happened because he did not wait the proper time, until his bowels had completely derived benefit from and had digested the articles taken at the preceding meal, and until his belly had become soft, and got into a state of rest, but he gave it a new supply while in a state of heat and fermentation, for such bellies digest much more slowly, and require more rest and ease. And as to him who had been accustomed to dinner, since, as soon as the body required food, and when the former meal was consumed, and he wanted refreshment, no new supply was furnished to it, he wastes and is consumed from want of food. For all the symptoms which I describe as befalling to this man I refer to want of food. And I also say that all men who, when in a state of health, remain for two or three days without food, experience the same unpleasant symptoms as those which I described in the case of him who had omitted to take dinner.

## Part XII

Wherefore, I say, that such constitutions as suffer quickly and strongly from errors in diet, are weaker than others that do not; and that a weak person is in a state very nearly approaching to one in disease; but a person in disease is the weaker, and it is, therefore, more likely that he should suffer if he encounters anything that is unseasonable. It is difficult, seeing that there is no such accuracy in the Art, to hit always upon what is most expedient, and yet many cases occur in medicine which would require this accuracy, as we shall explain. But on that account, I say, we ought not to reject the ancient Art, as if it were not, and had not been properly founded, because it did not attain accuracy in all things, but rather, since it is capable of reaching to the greatest exactitude by reasoning, to receive it and admire its discoveries, made from a state of great ignorance, and as having been well and properly made, and not from chance.

## Part XIII

But I wish the discourse to revert to the new method of those who prosecute their inquiries in the Art by hypothesis. For if hot, or cold, or moist, or dry, be that which proves injurious to man, and if the person who would treat him properly must apply cold to the hot, hot to the cold, moist to the dry, and dry to the moist- let me be presented with a man, not indeed one of a strong constitution, but one of the weaker, and let him eat wheat, such as it is supplied from the thrashing-floor, raw and unprepared, with raw meat, and let him drink water. By using such a diet I know that he will suffer much and severely, for he will experience pains, his body will become weak, and his bowels deranged, and he will not subsist long. What remedy, then, is to be provided for one so situated? Hot? or cold? or moist? or dry? For it is clear that it must be one or other of these. For, according to this principle, if it is one of the which is injuring the patient, it is to be removed by its contrary. But the surest and most obvious remedy is to change the diet which the person used, and instead of wheat to give bread, and instead of raw flesh, boiled, and to drink wine in addition to these; for by making these changes it is impossible but that he must get better, unless completely disorganized by time and diet. What, then, shall we say? whether that, as he suffered from cold, these hot things being applied were of use to him, or the contrary? I should think this question must prove a puzzler to whomsoever it is put. For whether did he who prepared bread out of wheat remove the hot, the cold, the moist, or the dry principle in it?- for the bread is consigned both to fire and to water, and is wrought with many things, each of which has its peculiar property and nature, some of which it loses, and with others it is diluted and mixed.

## Part XIV

And this I know, moreover, that to the human body it makes a great difference whether the bread be fine or coarse; of wheat with or without the hull, whether mixed with much or little water, strongly wrought or scarcely at all, baked or raw- and a multitude of similar differences; and so, in like manner, with the cake (maza); the powers of each, too, are great, and the one nowise like the other. Whoever pays no attention to these things, or, paying attention, does not comprehend them, how can he understand the diseases which befall a man? For, by every one of these things, a man is affected and changed this way or that, and the whole of his life is subjected to them, whether in health, convalescence, or disease. Nothing else, then, can be more important or more necessary to know than these things. So that the first inventors, pursuing their investigations properly, and by a suitable train of reasoning, according to the nature of man, made their discoveries, and thought the Art worthy of being ascribed to a god, as is the established belief. For they did not suppose that the dry or the moist, the hot or the cold, or any of these are either injurious to man, or that man stands in need of them, but whatever in each was strong, and more than a match for a man's constitution, whatever he could not manage, that they held to be hurtful, and sought to remove. Now, of the sweet, the strongest is that which is intensely sweet; of the bitter, that which is intensely bitter; of the acid, that which is intensely acid; and of all things that which is extreme, for these things they saw both existing in man, and proving injurious to him. For there is in man the bitter and the salt, the sweet and the acid, the sour and the insipid, and a multitude of other things having all sorts of powers both as regards quantity and strength. These, when all mixed and mingled up with one another, are not apparent, neither do they hurt a man; but when any of them is separate, and stands by itself, then it becomes perceptible, and hurts a man. And thus, of articles of food, those which are unsuitable and hurtful to man when administered, every one is either bitter, or intensely so, or saltish or acid, or something else intense and strong, and therefore we are disordered by them in like manner as we are by the secretions in the body. But all those things which a man eats and drinks are devoid of any such intense and well-marked quality, such as bread, cake, and many other things of a similar nature which man is accustomed to use for food, with the exception of condiments and confectioneries, which are made to gratify the palate and for luxury. And from those things, when received into the body abundantly, there is no disorder nor dissolution of the powers belonging to the body; but strength, growth, and nourishment result from them, and this for no other reason than because they are well mixed, have nothing in them of an immoderate character, nor anything strong, but the whole forms one simple and not strong substance.

## Part XV

I cannot think in what manner they who advance this doctrine, and transfer Art from the cause I have described to hypothesis, will cure men according to the principle which they have laid down. For, as far as I know, neither the hot nor the cold, nor the dry, nor the moist, has ever been found unmixed with any other quality; but I suppose they use the same articles of meat and drink as all we other men do. But to this substance they give the attribute of being hot, to that cold, to that dry, and to that moist. Since it would be absurd to advise the patient to take something hot, for he would straightway ask what it is? so that he must either play the fool, or have recourse to some one of the well known substances; and if this hot thing happen to be sour, and that hot thing insipid, and this hot thing has the power of raising a disturbance in the body (and there are many other kinds of heat, possessing many opposite powers), he will be obliged to administer some one of them, either the hot and the sour, or the hot and the insipid, or that which, at the same time, is cold and sour (for there is such a substance), or the cold and the insipid. For, as I think, the very opposite effects will result from either of these, not only in man, but also in a bladder, a vessel of wood, and in many other things possessed of far less sensibility than man; for it is not the heat which is possessed of great efficacy, but the sour and the insipid, and other qualities as described by me, both in man and out of man, and that whether eaten or drunk, rubbed in externally, and otherwise applied.

# Part XVI

But I think that of all the qualities heat and cold exercise the least operation in the body, for these reasons: as long time as hot and cold are mixed up with one another they do not give trouble, for the cold is attempered and rendered more moderate by the hot, and the hot by the cold; but when the one is wholly separate from the other, then it gives pain; and at that season when cold is applied it creates some pain to a man, but quickly, for that very reason, heat spontaneously arises in him without requiring any aid or preparation. And these things operate thus both upon men in health and in disease. For example, if a person in health wishes to cool his body during winter, and bathes either in cold water or in any other way, the more he does this, unless his body be fairly congealed, when he resumes his clothes and comes into a place of shelter, his body becomes more heated than before. And thus, too, if a person wish to be warmed thoroughly either by means of a hot bath or strong fire, and straightway having the same clothing on, takes up his abode again in the place he was in when he became congealed, he will appear much colder, and more disposed to chills than before. And if a person fan himself on account of a suffocating heat, and having procured refrigeration for himself in this manner, cease doing so, the heat and suffocation will be ten times greater in his case than in that of a person who does nothing of the kind. And, to give a more striking example, persons travelling in the snow, or otherwise in rigorous weather, and contracting great cold in their feet, their hands, or their head, what do they not suffer from inflammation and tingling when they put on warm clothing and get into a hot place? In some instances, blisters arise as if from burning with fire, and they do not suffer from any of those unpleasant symptoms until they become heated. So readily does either of these pass into the other; and I could mention many other examples. And with regard to the sick, is it not in those who experience a rigor that the most acute fever is apt to break out? And yet not so strongly neither, but that it ceases in a short time, and, for the most part, without having occasioned much mischief; and while it remains, it is hot, and passing over the whole body, ends for the most part in the feet, where the chills and cold were most intense and lasted longest; and, when sweat supervenes, and the fever passes off, the patient is much colder than if he had not taken the fever at all. Why then should that which so quickly passes into the opposite extreme, and loses its own powers spontaneously, be reckoned a mighty and serious affair? And what necessity is there for any great remedy for it?

## Part XVII

One might here say- but persons in ardent fevers, pneumonia, and other formidable diseases, do not quickly get rid of the heat, nor experience these rapid alterations of heat and cold. And I reckon this very circumstance the strongest proof that it is not from heat simply that men get into the febrile state, neither is it the sole cause of the mischief, but that this species of heat is bitter, and that acid, and the other saltish, and many other varieties; and again there is cold combined with other qualities. These are what proves injurious; heat, it is true, is present also, possessed of strength as being that which conducts, is exacerbated and increased along with the other, but has no power greater than what is peculiar to itself.

## Part XVIII

With regard to these symptoms, in the first place those are most obvious of which we have all often had experience. Thus, then, in such of us as have a coryza and defluxion from the nostrils, this discharge is much more acrid than that which formerly was formed in and ran from them daily; and it occasions swelling of the nose, and it inflames, being of a hot and extremely ardent nature, as you may know, if you apply your hand to the place; and, if the disease remains long, the part becomes ulcerated although destitute of flesh and hard; and the heat in the nose ceases, not when the defluxion takes place and the inflammation is present, but when the running becomes thicker and less acrid, and more mixed with the former secretion, then it is that the heat ceases. But in all those cases in which this decidedly proceeds from cold alone, without the concourse of any other quality, there is a change from cold to hot, and from hot to cold, and these quickly supervene, and require no coction. But all the others being connected, as I have said, with acrimony and intemperance of humors, pass off in this way by being mixed and concocted.

# Part XIX

But such defluxions as are determined to the eyes being possessed of strong and varied acrimonies, ulcerate the eyelids, and in some cases corrode the and parts below the eyes upon which they flow, and even occasion rupture and erosion of the tunic which surrounds the eyeball. But pain, heat, and extreme burning prevail until the defluxions are concocted and become thicker, and concretions form about the eyes, and the coction takes place from the fluids being mixed up, diluted, and digested together. And in defluxions upon the throat, from which are formed hoarseness, cynanche, crysipelas, and pneumonia, all these have at first saltish, watery, and acrid discharges, and with these the diseases gain strength. But when the discharges become thicker, more concocted, and are freed from all acrimony, then, indeed, the fevers pass away, and the other symptoms which annoyed the patient; for we must account those things the cause of each complaint, which, being present in a certain fashion, the complaint exists, but it ceases when they change to another combination. But those which originate from pure heat or cold, and do not participate in any other quality, will then cease when they undergo a change from cold to hot, and from hot to cold; and they change in the manner I have described before. Wherefore, all the other complaints to which man is subject arise from powers (qualities?). Thus, when there is an overflow of the bitter principle, which we call yellow bile, what anxiety, burning heat, and loss of strength prevail! but if relieved from it, either by being purged spontaneously, or by means of a medicine seasonably administered, the patient is decidedly relieved of the pains and heat; but while these things float on the stomach, unconcocted and undigested, no contrivance could make the pains and fever cease; and when there are acidities of an acrid and aeruginous character, what varieties of frenzy, gnawing pains in the bowels and chest, and inquietude, prevail! and these do not cease until the acidities be purged away, or are calmed down and mixed with other fluids. The coction, change, attenuation, and thickening into the form of humors, take place through many and various forms; therefore the crises and calculations of time are of great importance in such matters; but to all such changes hot and cold are but little exposed, for these are neither liable to putrefaction nor thickening. What then shall we say of the change? that it is a combination (crasis) of these humors having different powers toward one another. But the hot does not loose its heat when mixed with any other thing except the cold; nor again, the cold, except when mixed with the hot. But all other things connected with man become the more mild and better in proportion as they are mixed with the more things besides. But a man is in the best possible state when they are concocted and at rest, exhibiting no one peculiar quality; but I think I have said enough in explanation of them.

## Part XX

Certain sophists and physicians say that it is not possible for any one to know medicine who does not know what man is [and how he was made and how constructed], and that whoever would cure men properly, must learn this in the first place. But this saying rather appertains to philosophy, as Empedocles and certain others have described what man in his origin is, and how he first was made and constructed. But I think whatever such has been said or written by sophist or physician concerning nature has less connection with the art of medicine than with the art of painting. And I think that one cannot know anything certain respecting nature from any other quarter than from medicine; and that this knowledge is to be attained when one comprehends the whole subject of medicine properly, but not until then; and I say that this history shows what man is, by what causes he was made, and other things accurately. Wherefore it appears to me necessary to every physician to be skilled in nature, and strive to know, if he would wish to perform his duties, what man is in relation to the articles of food and drink, and to his other occupations, and what are the effects of each of them to every one. And it is not enough to know simply that cheese is a bad article of food, as disagreeing with whoever eats of it to satiety, but what sort of disturbance it creates, and wherefore, and with what principle in man it disagrees; for there are many other articles of food and drink naturally bad which affect man in a different manner. Thus, to illustrate my meaning by an example, undiluted wine drunk in large quantity renders a man feeble; and everybody seeing this knows that such is the power of wine, and the cause thereof; and we know, moreover, on what parts of a man's body it principally exerts its action; and I wish the same certainty to appear in other cases. For cheese (since we used it as an example) does not prove equally injurious to all men, for there are some who can take it to satiety without being hurt by it in the least, but, on the contrary, it is wonderful what strength it imparts to those it agrees with; but there are some who do not bear it well, their constitutions are different, and they differ in this respect, that what in their body is incompatible with cheese, is roused and put in commotion by such a thing; and those in whose bodies such a humor happens to prevail in greater quantity and intensity, are likely to suffer the more from it. But if the thing had been pernicious to of man, it would have hurt all. Whoever knows these things will not suffer from it.

## Part XXI

During convalescence from diseases, and also in protracted diseases, many disorders occur, some spontaneously, and some from certain things accidentally administered. I know that the common herd of physicians, like the vulgar, if there happen to have been any innovation made about that day, such as the bath being used, a walk taken, or any unusual food eaten, all which were better done than otherwise, attribute notwithstanding the cause of these disorders, to some of these things, being ignorant of the true cause but proscribing what may have been very proper. Now this ought not to be so; but one should know the effects of a bath or a walk unseasonably applied; for thus there will never be any mischief from these things, nor from any other thing, nor from repletion, nor from such and such an article of food. Whoever does not know what effect these things produce upon a man, cannot know the consequences which result from them, nor how to apply them.

## Part XXII

And it appears to me that one ought also to know what diseases arise in man from the powers, and what from the structures. What do I mean by this? By powers, I mean intense and strong juices; and by structures, whatever conformations there are in man. For some are hollow, and from broad contracted into narrow; some expanded, some hard and round, some broad and suspended, some stretched, some long, some dense, some rare and succulent, some spongy and of loose texture. Now, then, which of these figures is the best calculated to suck to itself and attract humidity from another body? Whether what is hollow and expanded, or what is solid and round, or what is hollow, and from broad, gradually turning narrow? I think such as from hollow and broad are contracted into narrow: this may be ascertained otherwise from obvious facts: thus, if you gape wide with the mouth you cannot draw in any liquid; but by protruding, contracting, and compressing the lips, and still more by using a tube, you can readily draw in whatever you wish. And thus, too, the instruments which are used for cupping are broad below and gradually become narrow, and are so constructed in order to suck and draw in from the fleshy parts. The nature and construction of the parts within a man are of a like nature; the bladder, the head, the uterus in woman; these parts clearly attract, and are always filled with a juice which is foreign to them. Those parts which are hollow and expanded are most likely to receive any humidity flowing into them, but cannot attract it in like manner. Those parts which are solid and round could not attract a humidity, nor receive it when it flows to them, for it would glide past, and find no place of rest on them. But spongy and rare parts, such as the spleen, the lungs, and the breasts, drink up especially the juices around them, and become hardened and enlarged by the accession of juices. Such things happen to these organs especially. For it is not with the spleen as with the stomach, in which there is a liquid, which it contains and evacuates every day; but when it (the spleen) drinks up and receives a fluid into itself, the hollow and lax parts of it are filled, even the small interstices; and, instead of being rare and soft, it becomes hard and dense, and it can neither digest nor discharge its contents: these things it suffers, owing to the nature of its structure. Those things which engender flatulence or tormina in the body, naturally do so in the hollow and broad parts of the body, such as the stomach and chest, where they produce rumbling noises; for when they do not fill the parts so as to be stationary, but have changes of place and movements, there must necessarily be noise and apparent movements from them. But such parts as are fleshy and soft, in these there occur torpor and obstructions, such as happen in apoplexy. But when it (the flatus?) encounters a broad and resisting structure, and rushes against such a part, and this happens when it is by nature not strong so as to be able to withstand it without suffering injury; nor soft and rare, so as to receive or yield to it, but tender, juicy, full of blood, and dense, like the liver, owing to its density and broadness, it resists and does not yield. But flatus, when it obtains admission, increases and becomes stronger, and rushes toward any resisting object; but owing to its tenderness, and the quantity of blood which it (the liver) contains, it cannot be without uneasiness; and for these reasons the most acute and frequent pains occur in the region of it, along with suppurations and chronic tumors (phymata). These symptoms also occur in the site of the diaphragm, but much less frequently; for the diaphragm is a broad, expanded, and resisting substance, of a nervous (tendinous?) and strong nature, and therefore less susceptible of pain; and yet pains and chronic abscesses do occur about it.

## Part XXIII

There are both within and without the body many other kinds of structure, which differ much from one another as to sufferings both in health and disease; such as whether the head be small or large; the neck slender or thick, long or short; the belly long or round; the chest and ribs broad or narrow; and many others besides, all which you ought to be acquainted with, and their differences; so that knowing the causes of each, you may make the more accurate observations.

## Part XXIV

And, as has been formerly stated, one ought to be acquainted with the powers of juices, and what action each of them has upon man, and their alliances towards one another. What I say is this: if a sweet juice change to another kind, not from any admixture, but because it has undergone a mutation within itself; what does it first become?- bitter? salt? austere? or acid? I think acid. And hence, an acid juice is the most improper of all things that can be administered in cases in which a sweet juice is the most proper. Thus, if one should succeed in his investigations of external things, he would be the better able always to select the best; for that is best which is farthest removed from that which is unwholesome.

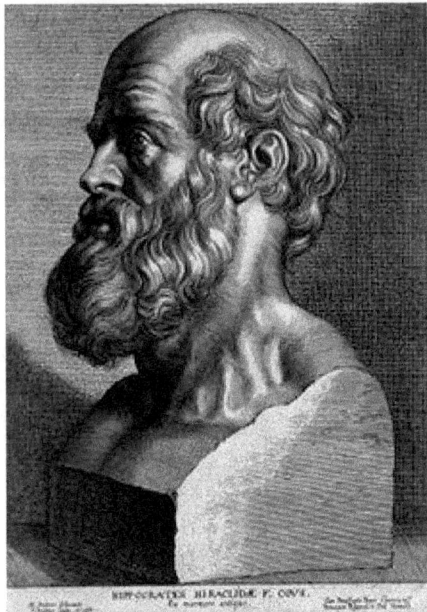

HIPPO'CRATES, the second of that name, and in some respects the most celebrated physician of ancient or modern times ; for not only have his writings (or rather those which bear his name) been always held in the highest esteem, but his personal history (so far as it is known), and the literary criticism relating to his works, furnish so much matter for the consideration both of the scholar, the philologist, the philosopher, and the man of letters, that there are few authors of antiquity about whom so much has been written. Probably the readers of this work will care more for the literary than for the medical questions connected with Hippocrates ; and accordingly (as it is quite impossible to discuss the whole subject fully in these pages) the strictly scientific portion of this article occupies less space than the critical ; and this arrangement in this place the writer is inclined to adopt the more readily, because, while there are many works which contain a good account of the scientific merits of the Hippocratic writings, he is not aware of one where the many literary problems arising from them have been at once fully discussed and satisfactorily determined. This task he is far from thinking that he has himself accomplished, but it is right to give this reason for treating the scientific part of the subject much less fully than he would have done had he been writing for a professed medical work.

A parallel has more than once been drawn be- tween " the Father of Medicine " and " the Father of Poetry ; " and, indeed, the resemblances between the two, both in their personal and literary historj', are so evident, that they could hardly fail to strike any one who was even moderately familiar with classical and medical literature. With respect to their personal history, the greatest uncertainty exists, and our real knowledge is next to nothing ; although in the case of both personages, we have professed lives written by ancient authors, which, however, only tend to show still more plainly the ignorance that prevails on the subject. Accordingly, as might be expected, fable has been busy in sup-plying the deficiencies of history, and was for a time fully believed ; till •sX length a re-action fol- lowed, and an unreasoning credulity was succeeded by an equally unreasonable scepticism, which reached its climax when it was boldly asserted that neither Homer nor Hippocrates had ever ex- istfid. (See Ilouclart, Etudes sur IJifypocrate^ p. 6G0.) The few facts respecting him that may be considered as tolerably well ascertained may be told in few words. His father was Ileracleides, who was also a physician, and belonged to the family of the Asclepiadae. According to Soraniis ( Vita Hippocr.^ in Ilippocr. Opera, vol. iii.), he was the nineteenth in descent from Aesculapius, but John Tzetzes, who gives the genealogy of the family, makes him the seventeenth. His niotlier's name was Phaenarete, who was said to be descended from Hercules. Soranus, on tlie autho- rity of an old writer who had composed a life of Hippocrates, states that he was born in the island of Cos, in the first year of the eightieth Olympiad, that is. B. c. 460 ; and this date is generally followed, for want of any more satisfactory inform- ation on the subject, though it agrees so ill with some of the anecdotes respecting him, that some persons suppose hira to have been born about thirty years sooner. The exact day of his birth was known and celebrated in Cos with sacrifices on the '26th. day of the month Agrianus,but it is unknown to what date in any other calendar this month cor- responds. He was instructed in medical science by his father and by Herodicus, and is also said to have been a pupil of Gorgias of Leontini. He wrote, taught, and practised his profession at home ; travelled in different parts of the continent of Greece ; and died at Larissa in Thessaly. His age at the time of his death is uncertain, as it is stated by different ancient authors to have been eighty-five years, ninety, one hundred and four, fend one hundred and nine. Mr. Clinton places his death B. c. 357, at the age of one hundred and four. He had two sons, Thessalus and Dracon, and a son-in-law, Polybus, all of whom followed the same profession, and who are supposed to have been the authors of some of the works in the Hippocratic Collection. Such are the few and scanty facts that can be in some degree depended on respecting the personal history of this cele- brated man ; but though we have not the means of writing an authentic detailed biography, we possess in these few facts, and in the hints and allusions con- tained in various ancient authors, sufficient data to enable us to appreciate the part he played, and the place he held among his contemporaries. We find that he enjoyed their esteem as a practitioner, writer, and professor; that he conferred on the ancient and illustrious family to which he belonged more honour than he derived from it ; that he rendered the medical school of Cos, to which he was attached, superior to any which had preceded it or immediately followed it ; and that his works, soon after their publication, were studied and quoted by Plato. (See Littre's Hippocr. vol. i. p. 43 ; and a review of that work (by the writer of this article) in the Brit, and For. Med. Rev. April, 1844, p. 459.)

Upon this slight foundation of historical truth has been built a vast superstructure of fabulous error ; and it is curious to observe how all these tales receive a colouring from the times and coun- tries in which they appear to have been fabricated, whether by his own countrymen before the Chris- tian era, or by the Latin or Arabic writers of the middle ages. One of the stories told of him by his Greek biograpners, which most modern critics are disposed to regard as fabulous, relates to his being sent for, together with Euryphon [EuRV- phon], by Perdiccas II., king of Macedonia, and discovering, by certain external symptoms, that his sickness was occasioned by his having fallen in love with his father's concubine. Probably the strongest reason against the truth of this story is the fact that the time of the supposed cure is quite irreconcileable with the commonly received date of the birth of Hippocrates ; though M. Litire, the latest and best editor of Hippocrates, while he rejects the story as spurious, finds no difficulty in the dates (vol. i. p. 38). Soranus, who tells tlie anecdote, says that the occurrence took place after the death of Alexander I., the father of Perdiccas; and we may rcasonabl} *presume that one or two* years would be the longest interval that would elapse. The date of the death of Alexander is not exactly known, and depends upon the length of the reign of his son Perdiccas, who died b. c. 414. The longest period assigned to his reign is forty- one years, the shortest is twenty-three. This latter date would place his accession to the throne on his father's death, at B. c. 437, at which time Hippo- crates would be only twenty-three years old, almost too young an age for him to have acquired so great celebrity as to be specially sent for to attend a foreign prince. However, the date of B. c. 437 is the less probable because it would not only extend the reign of his father Alexander to more than sixty years, but would also suppose him to have lived seventy years after a period at which he was already grown up to manhood. For these reasons Mr. Clinton {F. Hell. ii. 222 ) agrees with Dodwell in supposing the longer periods assigned to his reign to be nearer the truth ; and assumes the ac- cession of Perdiccas to have fallen within B. c. 454, at which time Hippocrates was only six years old. This celebrated story has been told, with more or less variation, of Erasistratus and Avicenna, besides being interwoven in the romance of Heliodorus (Aet/dop. iv, 7. p. 171), and the love-letters of Aristaenetus (Epist. i. 13). Galen also says that a similar circumstance happened to himself. (De Praenot. ad Epig. c. 6. vol. xiv. p. 630.) The story as applied to Avicenna seems to be most probably apocryphal (see Biogr. Diet, of the Usef. Knowl. Soc. vol. iv. p. 301) ; and with respect to the two other claimants, Hippocrates and Erasistratus, if it be true of either, the pre- ponderance of historical testimony is decidedly in favour of the latter. [Erasistratus.] Another old Greek fable relates to his being appointed librarian at Cos, and burning the books there (or, according to another version of the story, at Cnidos,) in order to conceal the use he had made of them in his own writings. This story is also told, with but little variation, of Avicenna, and is repeated of Hippocrates, with some characteristic embellish- ments, in the European Legends of the Middle Ages. [Andrkas.]

The other fables concerning Hippocrates are to be traced to the collection of Letters, &c. which go under his name, but which are universally rejected as spurious. The most celebrated of these relates to his supposed conduct during the plague of Athens, which he is said to have stopped by burn- ing fires throughout the city, by suspending chap- lets of flowers, and by the use of an antidote, the composition of which is preserved by Joannes Ac- tuarius {De Meth. Med. v. 6. p. 264, ed. H. Steph.) Connected with this, is the pretended letter from Artaxerxes Longimanus, king of Persia, to Hippocrates, inviting him by great offers to come to his assistance during a time of pestilence, and the re- fusal of Hippocrates, on the ground of his being the enemy of his country.

Another story, perhaps equally familiar to the readers of Burton's "Anatomy of Melancholy," contains the history of the supposed madness of Democritus, and his interview with Hippocrates, who had been sunnnoned by his countrymen to come to his relief.

If we turn to the Arabic writers, we find " Bokrdt " represented as living at Hems, and studying in a garden near Damascus, the situation of which was still pointed out in the time of Abu-1- faraj in the thirteenth century. (Abu-1-faraj, Hist. Dynast, p. 56; Anon. Arab. Philosoph. Bibl. apud Casiri, Bihlioth. A rahico-Hisp. Escur. vol. i. p. 235.) They also tell a story of his pupils taking his por- trait to a celebrated physiognomist named Phile- mon., in order to try his skill ; and that upon his saying that it was the portrait of a lascivious old man ( which they strenuously denied), Hippocrates said that he was right, for that he was so by nature, but that he had learned to overcome his amorous propensities. The confusion of names that occurs in this last anecdote the writer has never seen explained, though the difficulty admits of an easy and satisfactory solution. It will no doubt have brought to the reader's recollection the similar story told of Socrates by Cicero (Tusc. Disp. iv. 37, De Fata., c. 5), and accordingly he will be quite prepared to hear that the Arabic writers have confounded the word ]b^ JL«j Sokrut^ with ^^ Jj Boki-at., and have thus applied to Hippocrates an anecdote that in reality belongs to Socrates. The name of the physiognomist in Cicero is Zopyrus, which cannot have been corrupted into Philemon ; but when we remember that the Arabians have no /*, and are therefore often obliged to express this letter by an F^ it will probably appear not unlikely that either the writers, or their European trans- lators, have confounded Philemon with Polemon. This conjecture is confirmed by the fact that Phile- mon is said by Abu-1-faraj to have written a work on Physiognomy, which is true of Polemon, whose treatise on that subject is still extant, whereas no person of the name of Philemon (as far as the writer is aware) is mentioned as a physiognomist by any Greek author.* The only objection to this conjecture is the anachronism of making Pole- mon a contemporary of Hippocrates or Socrates ; but this difficulty will not appear very great to any one who is familiar with the extreme igno- rance and carelessness displayed by the Arabic writers on all points of Greek history and chro- nology.

It is, however, among the European story- tellers of the middle ages that the name of " Ypo- cras " is most celebrated. In one story he is repre- sented as visiting Rome during the reign of Au- gustus, and restoring to life the emperor's nephew, who was just dead ; for which service Augustus

- There is at this present time among the MSS.

at Leyden a little Arabic treatise on Physiognomy which bears the name of Philemon., and which (as the writer has been informed by a gentleman who has compared the two works) bears a very great resemblance to the Greek treatise by Polemon. {JXQ Catal. Biblioth. Lujdun. p. 461. § 1286.)

erected a statue in his honour as to a divinity. A fair lady resolved to prove that this god was a mere mortal ; and, accordingly, having made an assignation with him, she let down for him a basket from her window. When she had raised him half way, she left him suspended in the air all night, till he was found by the emperor in the morning, and thus became the laughing-stock of the court. Anoiher story makes him professor of medicine in Rome, with a nephew of wondrous talents and medical skill, whom he despatched in his own stead to the king of Hungary, who had sent for him to heal his son. The young leech, by his marvellous skill, having discovered that the prince was not the king's own son, directed him to feed on " contrarius drink, contrarius mete, beves flesch, and drink the broth t," and thereby soon restored him to health. Upon his return home laden with presents, " Ypocras" became so jealous of his fame, that he murdered him, and afterwards " he let all his bokes berne." The vengeance of Heaven overtook him, and he died in dreadful torments, confessing his crime, and vainly calling on his murdered nephew for relief. (See Ellis, Spec, of Early Engl. Metr. Roman, vol. iii. p. 39 ; Weber, Metr. Rom. of the Wi, Uh, and bth Cent.., ^c, vol. iii. p. 41 ; Way, Fabliaux or Talcs of the ih and 'Mh Cent.^ ^c. vol. ii. p. 173 ; Le- grand d'Aussy, Fabliaux ou Contes, Fables et Ro- mans du eme et du ?>eme Siecles, tome i. p. 288 ; Loiseleur Deslongchamps, Essai sur les Fables Ind. ^c, p. 154, and Roman des Sept Sages, p. 26.)

If, from the personal history of Hippocrates, we turn to the collection of writings that go under his name, the parallel with Homer will be still more exact and striking. In both cases we find a number of works, the most ancient, and, in some respects, the most excellent of their kind, which, though they have for centuries borne the same name, are discovered, on the most cursory examination, to belong in reality to several different persons. Hence has arisen a question which has for ages exercised the learning and acuteness of scholars and critics, and which is in both cases still far from being satisfactorily settled. With respect to the writings of the Hippocratic Collection " the first glance," says M. Littre (vol. i. p. 44), *' shows that some are complete in themselves, while others are merely collections of notes, which follow each other without connection, and which are sometimes hardly intelligible. Some are incomplete and fragmentary, others form in the whole Collection particular series, which belong to the same ideas and the same writer. In a word, however little we reflect ou the context of these numerous writings, we are led to conclude that they are not the work of one and the same author. This remark has in all ages struck those persons who have given their atten- tion to the works of Hippocrates ; and even at the time when men commented on them in the Alex- andrian school, they already disputed about their authenticity."

But it is not merely from internal evidence (though this of itself would be sufficiently con- vincing) that we find that the Hippocratic Collec- tion is not the work of Hippocrates alone, for it so happens that in two insUinces we find a passage that has appeared from very early times as forming part of this collection, quoted as belonging to a dilfereut person. Indeed if we had nothing but internal evidence to guide us in our task of ex- amining these writings, in order to decide which really belong to Hippocrates, we should come to but few positive results ; and therefore it is neces- sary to collect all the ancient testimonies that can still be found ; in doing which, it will appear that the Collection, as a whole, can be traced no higher than the period of the Alexandrian school, in the third century b. c. ; but that particular treatises are referred to by the contemporaries of Hippocrates and his immediate successors. {^Brit. and For. Med. Rev. p. 460.)

We find that Hippocrates is mentioned or re- ferred to by no less than ten persons anterior to the foundation of the Alexandrian school, and among them by Aristotle and Plato. At the time of the formation of the great Alexandrian library, the different treatises which bear the name of Hip- pocrates were diligently sought for, and formed into a single collection ; and about this time commences the series of Commentators, which has continued through a period of more than two thousand years to the present day. The first person who is known to have commented on any of the works of the Hippocratic Collection is Herophilus. [Herophi- Lus.] The most ancient commentary still in ex- istence is that on the treatise " De Articulis," by ApoUonius Citiensis. [Apollonius Citiensis.] By far the most voluminous, and at the same time by far the most valuable commentaries that remain, are those of Galen, who wrote several works in illustration of the writings of Hippocrates, besides those which we now possess. His Commentaries, which are still extant, are those on the " De Na- tura Hominis," " De Salubri Victus Ratione," " De Ratione Victus in Morbis Acutis," " Praenotiones," " Praedictiones I.," " Aphorismi," " De Morbis Vulgaribus I. II. III. VI," " De Fracturis," "De Articulis," " De OfRcina Medici," and " De Hu- moribus," with a glossary of difficult and obsolete words, and fragments on the " De Aere, Aquis, et Locis," and " De Alimento." The other ancient commentaries that remain are those of Palladius, Joannes Alexandrinus, Stephanus Atheniensis, Meletius, Theophilus Protospatharius, and Damas- cius ; besides a spurious work attributed to Ori- basius, a glossary of obsolete and difficult words by I'lrotianus, and some Arabic Commentaries that have never been published. {^Brit. and For. Med. Rev. p. 461.)

His writings were held in the highest esteem by the ancient Greek and Latin physicians, and most of them were translated into Arabic. (See Wen- rich, De Auct. Grace. Vers, et Comment. Syr. Arab., &c.) In the middle ages, however, they were not so much studied as those of some other authors, whose works are of a more practical cha- racter, and better fitted for being made a class-book and manual of instruction. In more modern times, on the contrary, the works of the Hippocratic Col- lection have been valued more according to their real worth, while many of the most popular medical writers of the middle ages have fallen into complete neglect. The number of works written in illustra- tion or explanation of the Collection is very great, as is also that of the editions of the whole or any part ol the treatises composing it. Of these only a very few can be here mentioned : a fuller account may be found in Fabric. Bibl. Grace. ; Haller, Bibl. Medic. Pract.; the first vol. of Kiihn's edi- tion of Hippocrates; Choulanfs Ilandb. der Bu- clierTcunde fur die Aellere Medicin ; Littre's Hip- pocrates ; and other professed bibliographical works. 'J'he works of Hippocrates first appeared in a Latin translation by Fabius Calvus, Rom. 1525, fol. The first Greek edition is the Aldine, Venet. 1526, fol., which was printed from MSS. with hardly any correction of the transcriber's errors. The first edition that had any pretensions to be called a critical edition was that by Hieron. Mercurialis, Venet. 1588, fol., Gr. and Lat. ; but this was much surpassed by that of Anut. Foesius, Francof. 1595, fol., Gr. and Lat., which continues to the present day to be the best complete edition. Van- der Linden's edition (Lugd. Bat. 1 665, 8vo. 2 vols. Gr. and Lat.) is neat and commodious for refer- ence from his having divided the text into short paragraphs. Chartier's edition of the works of Galen and Hippocrates has been noticed under Galen; as has also Kiihn's, of which it may be said that its only advantages are its convenient size, the reprint of Ackermann's Histor. Liter. Hippocr. (from Harless's ed. of Fabr. Bibl. Gr.) in the first vol., and the noticing on each page the cor- responding pagination of the editions of Foes, Chartier, and Vander Linden. By far the best edition in every respect is one which is now in the course of publication at Paris, under the super- intendence of E. Littre, of which the first vol. ap- peared in 1839, and the fourth in 1844. It contains a new text, founded upon a collation of the MSS. in the Royal Library at Paris ; a French translation ; an interesting and learned general In- troduction, and a copious argument prefixed to each treatise ; and numerous scientific and philological notes. It is a work quite indispensable to every physician, critic, and philologist, who wishes to study in detail the works of the Hippocratic Col- lection, and it has already done much more to- wards settling the text than any edition that has preceded it ; but at the same time it must not be concealed that the editor does not seem to have always made the best use of the materials that he has had at his command, and that the classical reader cannot help now and then noticing a mani- fest want of critical (and even at times of gram- matical) scholarship.

The Hippocratic Collection consists of more than sixty works ; and the classification of these, and assigning each (as far as possible) to its proper author, constitutes by far the most diffi- cult question connected with the ancient medical writers. Various have been the classifications proposed both in ancient and modem times, and various the rules by which their authors were guided ; some contenting themselves with following implicitly the opinions of Galen and Erotianus, others arguing chiefly from peculiarities of style, while a tliird class distinguished the books accord- ing to the medical and philosophical doctrines contained in them. An account of each of these classifications cannot be given here, much less can the objections that may be brought against each be pointed out : upon the whole, the writer is inclined to think M. Littre's superior to any that has pre- ceded it ; but by no means so imexceptionable as to do away with the necessity of a new one. The following classification, though far enough from supplying the desideratum, difi'ers in several in- stances from any former one : it is impossible here for the writer to give more than the results of his investigation, referring for the data on which hia opinion in each particular case is founded to the works of Gniner, Ackermann, and Littre, of which he has, of course, made free use.* Perhaps a tabular or genealogical view of the different divisions and subdivisions of the Collection will be the best cal- culated to put the reader at once in possession of the whole bearings of the subject.

The Hippocratic Collection consists of Works certainltf ■written by Hip- pocrates. (Class Works certainly not written by Hippocrates. Works perhaps written by Hip- pocrates. (Class ll.) Works earliei than Hippo- crates. (Class III.) Works later than Hippo- crates. Works about contemporary with Hippo- crates. I >Vorks authentic, but not genuine, i. e. not wilful forgeries. Works neither genuine nor authentic, i.e. wilful forge- ries. (Class VIII.) I I Works whose Works whose author is author is conjectured. unknown. (Class IV.) (Class V.) Works by va- rious authors. (Class VII.) Works by the same author. (Class VI.)

Class I., containing UpoyuaxTTiKdv, Praenotiones or Prognosticon (vol. i. p. 88, ed. Kiihn) ; 'A^o- pia-fiol, Aphorismi (vol. iii. p. 706) ; 'EiridTjixicou Bi§ia A, r, De Morbis Popularilms (or Epidemi- orum lib. i. and iii. (vol. i. pp. 382, 467) ; Hept AjaiTTjs 'O|6oj]', De Ratione Victus in Morbis Acutis, or De Diaeta Acutorum (vol. ii. p. 25); Tlepi *Aepiou^ 'TSdruv^ Tottwv, De Acre, Aquisy et Locis (vol. i. p, 523) ; Uepl twu kv KecpoKfj Tpu- ixdruu, De Capitis Vulneribus (vol. iii. p. 346).

Class II., containing Ilepl "Apxaf-ns 'iTjTpj/crjy, De Prisca Medidna (vol. i. p. 22) ; Hep! "Apdpwv, De Articidis (vol. iii. p. 135); Uepl ^KyixSv^ De Fradis (vol. iii. p. 64); MoxA.tKos, MochUms or Vectiarius (vol. iii. p. 270) ; "OpKos, Jicsjurandum (vol. i. p. 1) ; ^o/xos. Lex (vol. i. p. 3); Ilepl 'E/c(Sj', De Ulceribus (vol. iii. p. 307) ; Tl^pX ^vpiyywv^ De Fistulis (vol. iii. p. 329); Uepl AtfjLo^pot^cov^ De Haemorrhoidibus (o. iii. p. 340); KaT* 'iTjrpetoj', De Officina Medici (vol. iii. p. 48) ; TlepX 'Iprjs Uovaov^ De Morbo Sacra (vol. i. p. 587).

Class III., containing Tlpo^f)7}riK6v A, Pror- rlietica^ or Praedidiones i. (vol. i. p. 157) ; KcoaKot npoyvdaeis, Coacae Praenotiones (vol. i. p. 234).

Class IV., containing Uspl ^vcrios 'Avdpciirov, De Natura Hominis (vol. i. p. 348) ; riepl Aiairrts "Tyieivrjs, De Salubri Victus Ratione {?) (vol. i. p. 616); riepl TouaiK^i-n^ ^uaios, De Natura Mu- liebri(?) (vol. ii. p. 529) ; Uepl Nomwv B, T, De Morbis, ii. iii(?) (volii. p.212); Uepl 'EmKv^<rios, De Super/oetatione{?) (vol. i. p. 460).

Class v., containing Uepl Ouawi', De Phtibus (vol. i. p. 569) ; Uepl TSituv twv kut "AvOpwrrov^ De Locis in Homine (vol. ii. p. 101) ; Ilepl Texi'Tjy, De Arte{?) (vol. i. p. 5) ; Uepl AiatTijs, De Diaeta, or De Victus Ratione (vol. i. p. 625) ; Uepl 'Ei/u-

- Some of the readers of this work may perhaps

be interested to hear that a strictly ;)A«7o/or/2ca/ clas- sification of the works of the Hippocratic Collection is still a desideratum ; and that, as this is in fact almost the only question connected with the subject which has not by this time been thoroughly ex- amined, any scholar who will undertake the work will be doing good service to the cause of ancient medical literature.

■npltav, De Insomniis (vol. ii. p. 1); Uepl UaOwv, De Affectionibus (vol. ii. p. 380) ; Uepl tcov evros UadoSu, De Internis Affectionilms (vol. ii. p. 427) ; Uepl Novaav A, De Morbis i. (vol. ii. p. 1 65 ) ; Uepl 'EirTajj-riuov, De Septimestri Partu (vol. i. p. 444) ; Uepl 'OKTafxrivov, De Octimestri Partu (vol. i. p. 455) ; ^EiTi8'r]ixi(av Bi§la B, A, Z, Epidemiorum, or De Morbis Popularibtis, ii. iv. vi. (vol. iii. pp. 428, 511, 583) ; Uepl Xv/jlu/v, De Ilumoribus (vol. i. p. 120) ; Uepl 'Typwv Xpijaios, De Usu Liqui- dorum (vol. ii. p. 153).

Class VI., containing Uepl Vovrs, De Genitura (vol. i. p. 371) ; Uepl ^va-ios UaiSiov, De Natura Pueri (vol. i. p. 382) ; Ilepl 'No^awv A, De Morbis iv. (vol. ii. p. 324) ; Uepl TuvaiKeim', De Mu- lierum Morbis (vol. ii. p. 606) ; Utpl Uap6ei>iw}/, De Virginum Morbis (vol. ii. p. 526) ; Uepl 'A(p6- puiv, De Sterilibus (vol. iii. p. 1).

Class VII., containing 'EttjStJjUiwi' BigAta E, H, Epidemiorum, or De Morbis Popularibus v. vii. fvol. iii. pp. 545, 631) ; UeX KapStTjy, De Corde (vol. i. p. 485) ; Ilept Tpo<pT/s, De Alimento (vol. ii. p. 17) ; Ilept ^dpKoou, De Carnibus (vol. i. p. 424); Uepl 'ESSofjidSuv, De Septimanis, a work which no longer exists in Greek, but of which M. Littr6 has found a Latin translation ; Upop^rjTiKou B, Prorrhetica (or

Praedidiones) ii. (vol. i. p. 185) ; Uepl 'Oa-Tewu ^vcrios, De Natura Ossium, a work composed entirely of extracts from other treatises of the Hippocratic Collection, and from other an- cient authors, and which therefore M. Littre is going to suppress entirely ( vol. i. p. 502) ; Uepl 'ASevwu, De Glandtdis (vol. i. p. 491); Uepl 'iTjTpov, De Medico (vol. i. p. 56) ; Uepl Ev- o'XVfJ-oavvTjs, De Decenti Habitu (vol. i. p. 66) ; UapayyeXiai, Praeceptiones (vol. i. p. 77) ; Uepl 'AvaTopLris, De Anatomia (or De Resedione Cor- porum) (vol. iii. p. 379) ; Uepl 'OSourocpvi'-ns, De Dmtitione (vol. i. p. 482) ; Uepl ^Ey Kararojxris 'E/i- Spvov, De Resedione Foetus (vol. iii. p. 376) ; Uepl "Oxl/ios, De Visu (vol. iii. p. 42) ; Uepl Kpialcau, De Crisibus (or De Judicationibus) (vol. i. p. 136) ; Uepl Kpiaifxwu, De Diebus Criticis (or De Diebus Judicatortis) (vol. i. p. 149) ; Uepl ^apixoLKoav, De Medicamentis Purgativis (vol. iii. p. 855 j.

Class VIII., containing 'EtnaroKal, Epistolae (vol. iii. p. 769) ; UpecrSevrinos ©eaaaXou, Tlies- sali Legati Oratio (vol. iii. p. 831); 'Etv iSoifxios, Oratio ad Aram (vol. iii. p. 830) ; Aoyjxa 'AOrj- vaicov, Atlieniensium Senatus Consultum (vol. iii. p. 829).

Each of these classes requires a few words of explanation. The first class will probably be con- sidered by many persons to be rather small ; but it seemed safer and better to include in it only those works of whose genuineness there has never been any doubt. To this there is perhaps one ex- ception, and that relating to the very work whose genuineness one would perhaps least expect to find called in question, as it is certainly that by which Hippocrates is most popularly known. Some doubts have arisen in the minds of several eminent critics as to the origin of the Aphorisms, and indeed the discussion of the genuineness of this work may be said to be an epitome of the questions relating to the whole Hippocratic Collection. We find here a very celebrated work, which has from early times borne the name of Hippocrates, but of which some parts have always been condemned as spurious. Upon examining tliose portions that are considered to be genuine, we observe that the greater part of the first three sections agrees almost word for word with passages to be found in his acknowledged works ; while in the remaining sections we find sentences fciken apparently from spurious or doubt- ful treatises ; thus adding greatly to our difficulties, inasmuch as they sometimes contain doctrines and theories opposed to those which we find in the works acknowledged to be genuine. And these facts are (in the opinion of the critics alluded to) to be accounted for in one of two ways : either Hippocrates himself in his old age (for the Apho- risms have always been attributed to this period of his life) put together certain extracts from his own works, to which were afterwards added other sen- tences taken from later authors ; or else the col- lection was not formed by Hippocrates himself, but by some person or persons after his death, who made aphoristical extracts from his works, and from those of other writers of a later date, and the whole was then attributed to Hippocrates, because he was the author of the sentences that were most valuable, and came first in order. This account of the formation of the Aphorisms appears extremely plausible, nor does it seem to be any decisive ob- jection to say, that we find among them sentences which are not to be met with elsewhere ; for, when we recollect how many works of the old medical writers, and perhaps of Hippocrates himself, are lost, it is easy to conceive that these sentences may have been extracted from some treatise that is no longer in existence. It must however be con- fessed that this conjecture, however plausible and probable, requires further proof and examination before it can be received as true.

The second class is one of the most unsatisfac- tory in the writers own opinion, and affords at the same time a curious instance of the impossibility of satisfying even those few persons in Europe whose opinion on such a matter is really worth asking ; fi)r, upon submitting the classification to two friends, one of whom is decidedly the most learned phy- sician in Great Britain, and the other one of the best medical critics on the continent, he was ad- vised by the one to call this class "Works probably written by Hippocrates," and by the other to trans- fer them (with one exception) to the class of

- ' Works certainly not written by Hippocrates."

The amount of probability in favour of the genuine- ness of all these works is certainly by no means equal ; e. g. the two little pieces called the " Oath," and thS " Law," though commonly considered to be the work of the same author, and to be in- timately connected with each other, seem rather to belong to different periods, the former having all the simplicity, honesty, and religious feeling of an- tiquity, the latter somewhat of the affectation and declamatory grandiloquence of a sophist. How- ever, as all of these books have been considered to be genuine by some critics of more or less note, it seemed better to defer to their authority at least 80 far as to allow that they might perhaps have been written by Hippocrates himself.

The two works which constitute the third class, and which are probably the oldest medical writings that exist, have been supposed with some proba- bility to consist, at least in part, of the inscriptions on the votive tablets placed in the temple of Aescu- lapius by those who had recovered their health, which certJiinly constituted one of the sources from which the medical knowledge of Hippocrates was derived.

In the fourth class are placed those works which were certainly not written by Hippocrates himself, which were probably either contemporary or but little posterior to him, and whose authors have been, with more or less degree of certainty, dis- covered. The works De Natura Hoini/ns, and I)e Salubri Victus Ratmie^ are supposed by M. Littre to have been written by the same author, because it is said by Galen that in many old editions these two treatises formed but one ; and this author he concludes to have been Polybus, the son-in-law of Hippocrates (vol. i. pp. 46, 316, &c.), because a passage is quoted by Aristotle {Hist. Aiiiin. .iii ?>), and attributed to Polybus, which is found word for word in the work De Natura Iluminis (vol. i. p. 364). For somewhat similar reasons, Euryphon has been supposed to be the author of the second and third books De Morbis, and the work De Natura Muliebri [Euryphon] ; and also (though with much less show of reason) a certain Leo- phanes, or Cleophanes (of whom nothing whatever is known), to have written the treatise De Sujxrr- foetatione (Littr^, vol. i p. 380).

In the fifth class there is one treatise {De Di- aeta) in which an astronomical, coincidence with the calendar of Eudoxus has been pointed to the writer by a friend, which (as far as he is aware) has never been noticed by any commentator on Hippocrates, and which seems in some degree to fix the date of the work in question. If the ca- lendar of Eudoxus, as preserved in the Ajyparentiae of Ptolemy and the calendar of Geminus (see Petav. Uranol. pp. 64, 71), be compared with part of the third book De Diaeta (vol. i. pp. 7 1 1 —7 1 5 ), it will be found that the periods correspond so exactly, that (there being no other solar calendar of antiquity in which these intervals coincide so closely,and all through,but that of Eudoxus), it seems a reasonable inference that the writer of the work De Diaeta took them from the calendar in question. If this be granted, it will follow that the author must have written this work after the year B. c. 381, which is the date of the calendar of Eu- doxus ; and, as Hippocrates must have been at least eighty years old at that time, this conclusion will agree quite well with the general opinion of ancient and modern critics, that the treatise in question was probably written by one of his im- mediate followers.

The sixth class agrees with the sixth class of M. Littr^, who, with great appearance of proba- bility, supposes it to form a connected series of works written by the same author, whose name is quite unknown, and of whose date it can only be determined from internal evidence that he must have lived later than Hippocrates, and before the time of Aristotle.

The works contained in this and the seventh class have for many centuries formed part of the Hippocratic Collection without having any right to such an honour, and therefore are not genuine ; but, as it does not appear that their authors were guilty of assuming the name of Hippocrates, or that they have represented the state of medical science as in any respect different from what it really was in the times in which they wrote, there is no reason for denying their authenticity. And in this respect they are to be regarded with a very different eye from the pieces which form the last class, which are neither genuine nor authentic, but mere forgeries ; which display indeed here and there some ingenuity and skill, but which are still sufficiently full of difficulties and inconsistencies to betray at once their origin.

So much space has been taken up with the pre- liminary, but most indispensable step of determin- ing which are the genuine works of Hippocrates, and which are spurious, that a very slight sketch of his opinions is all that can be now attempted, and for a fuller account the reader must be referred to the works of Le Clerc, Haller, Sprengel, &c., or to some of those which relate especially to Hippo- crates, He divides the causes of disease into two principal classes ; the one comprehending the in- fluence of seasons, climates, water, situation, &c., and the other consisting of more personal and pri- vate causes, such as result from the particular kind and amount of food and exercise in which each separate individual indulges himself. The modifi- cations of the atmosphere dependent on different seasons and climates is a subject which was suc- cessfully treated by Hippocrates, and which is still far from exhausted by all the researches of modern science. He considered that while heat and cold, moisture and dryness, succeeded one another throughout the year, the human body underwent certain analogous changes, which influenced the diseases of the period ; and on this basis was founded the doctrine of pathological constitutions, corresponding to particular conditions of the at- mosphere, so that, whenever the year or the season exhibited a special character in which such or such a temperature prevailed, those persons who were exposed to its influence were affected by a series of disorders, all bearing the same stamp. (How plainly the same idea runs through the Observaii- ones Medicae of Sydenham, our *English Hippo-crates* " need not be pointed out to those who are at all familiar with his works.) Tlie belief in the influence which different climates exercise on the human frame follows naturally from the theory just mentioned ; for, in fact, a climate may be con- sidered as nothing more than a permanent season, whose effects may be expected to be more power-ful, inasmuch as the cause is ever at work upon mankind. Accordingly, Hippocrates attributes to climate both the conformation of the body and the disposition of the mind — indeed, almost every thing ; and if the Greeks were found to be hardy freemen, and the Asiatics effeminate slaves, he accounts for the difference of their characters by that of the climates in which they lived. With respect to the second class of causes producing disease, he attributed all sorts of disorders to a vicious system of diet, which, whether excessive or defective, he considered to be equally injurious ; and in the same way' he supposed that, when bo- dily exercise was either too much indulged in or entirely neglected, the health was equally likely to suffer, thougli by different forms of disease. Into all the minutiae of the " Humoral Pathology " (as it was called), which kept its ground in FJurope as the prevailing doctrine of all the medical sects for more than twenty centuries, it would be out of place to enter here. It will be sufficient to remind the reader that the four fluids or humours of the body (blood, phlegm, yellow bile, and black bile) were supposed to be the primary seat of disease ; that health was the result of the due combination (or crash) of these, and that, when this crasis was disturbed, disease was the consequence ; that, iu the course of a disorder that was proceeding fa-vourably, these humours underwent a certain change in quality (or coction), which was the sign of returning health, as preparing the way for the expulsion of the morbid matter, or crisis; and that these crises had a tendency to occur at certain stated periods, which were hence called " critical days." {Brit, and For. Med. Rev.)

The medical practice of Hippocrates was cautious and feeble, so much so, that he was in after times reproached with letting his patients die, by doing nothing to keep them alive. It consisted chiefly in watching tiie operations of nature, and pro- moting the critical evacuations mentioned above ; so that attention to diet and regimen was the principal and often the only remedy that he em- ployed. Several hundred substances have been enumerated which are used medicinally in different parts of the Hippocratic Collection ; of these, by far the greater portion belong to the vegetable kingdom, as it would be in vain to look for any traces of chemistry in these early writings. In surgery, he is the author of the frequently quoted maxim, that " what cannot be cured by medicines is cured by the knife ; and what cannot be cured by the knife is cured by fire." The anatomical knowledge displayed in different parts of the Hip- pocratic Collection is scanty and contradictory, so much so, that the discrepancies on this subject constitute an important criterion in deciding the genuineness of the different treatises.

With regard to the personal character of Hip- pocrates, though he says little or nothing expressly about himself, yet it is impossible to avoid drawing certain conclusions from the characteristic passages scattered through the pages of his writings. He was evidently a person who not only had had great experience, but who also knew how to turn it to the best account ; and the number of moral reflections and apophthegms that we meet with in his writings, some of which (as, for example, " Life is short, and Art is long ") have acquired a sort of proverbial notoriety, show him to have been a profound thinker. He appears to have felt the moral obligations and responsibilities of his profession, and often tries to impress upon his readers the duties of care and attention, and kind- ness towards the sick, saying that a physician's first and chief consideration ought to be the re- storing his patient to health. The style of the Hippocratic writings, which are in the Ionic dialect, is so concise as to be sometimes extremely ohscure ; though this charge, which is as old as the time of Galen, is often brought too indiscriminately against the whole collection, whereas it applies, in fact especially only to certain treatises, which seem to be merely a collection of notes, such as De IJu- moribiis, De Alimeido^ De Ojjlcina Medici, &c. In those writings, which are universally allowed to be genuine, we do not find this excessive brevity, though even these are in general by no means easy. {Brit, and For. Med. Rev. )

Of the great number of books published on the subject of the Hippocratic Collection, only a very few of the most modern and most useful can be here enumerated ; a fuller list may be found in Choulant's Handb. der li'ucherkunde fur die Aeltere Medicin, or his Biblioth. Medico- 1 Hi- tor. ; or in Ackermann's Historia Literaria Ilijypo- crutis. Fiiesii Oeco7iomia Ilippocrads is a very copious and learned lexicon, published in fol. Francof. 1588, and Gene v. I(i62. Sprengel'B Apologie des Hippocr. und seiner Grundsatze (Leipz. 1789, 1792, 2 vols. 8vo.), contains, among other matter, a Gennan translation of some of tlie genuine treatises, with a valuable commentary. The treatise by Ermerins, De Hippocr. Doctrina a Prognostice oriunda (Lugd. Bat. 1832, 4to,), de- serves to be carefully studied ; as also does Link's dissertation, Ueher die Theorien in den Hippocra- tisclien Schriften^ nebst Bemerkungen uber die Echt- I/eit dieser ScJinflen^ in the * *Abhandlungen der* Berlin. Akadem.*' 1814, 1815. Gruner's Censura Lil)rorum Hippocraieorum qua veri a fulsis^ intcgri a supj)ositis segreganiur, Vratislav. 1772, 8vo., con- tains a useful account of the amount of evidence in favour of each treatise of the collection, though his conclusions are not always to be depended on. See al«o Houdart, Etudes Histor. et Crit. sur la Vie et kc Doctrine d' Hippocr. Paris, 183G, 8vo.; Petersen, Hippocr. Nomine quae circuiiiferuntur Scripta ad Temporis Raiiones dispos. Hamburg, 1839, 4to. ; Meixner, Neue Prnfung der Eehtlieit und Reiliefolge S'dmmtlicher Schriften Hippocr.^ Miinchen, 1836, 1837, 8vo. [W. A. G.]

www.ingramcontent.com/pod-product-compliance
Lightning Source LLC
Chambersburg PA
CBHW071532210326
41597CB00018B/2971